Heart healthy cookbook for all for all

Easy Delicious, Low Fat, Low Sodium
Heart Healthy Recipes

Donald Turner

Copyright Statement © 2024 Donald Turner

While every effort has been made to ensure the accuracy and reliability of the information in this cookbook, the author and publisher disclaim responsibility for any adverse effects resulting directly or indirectly from the use of the recipes or advice provided. Readers are advised to consult with healthcare professionals for personalized guidance on their dietary choices and health concerns.

Table Of Contents

INTRODUCTION

Welcome to Heart healthy cookbook for all

In the rhythmic tapestry of our lives, the heartbeat serves as a constant reminder of the vitality that courses through our veins. This cookbook, "Heart healthy cookbook for all: Easy Delicious, Low Fat, Low Sodium Heart Healthy Recipes," is not just a compilation of culinary creations; it is a story—a narrative woven with the threads of health, flavor, and a deep understanding of the intricate dance our hearts perform each day.

Our journey begins with a personal tale, one that inspired the creation of Heart healthy cookbook for all. A few years ago, our founder, Jane, found herself at a crossroads when her doctor shared concerns about her heart health. Faced with this pivotal moment, she embarked on a quest to not only nourish her body but also to mend and protect her most vital organ—the heart.

Through research, consultations, and the guidance of nutritionists, Jane discovered the power of heart-friendly eating. This cookbook is a testament to her transformative journey, showcasing the delicious and nutrient-rich recipes that not only revitalized her health but also became a beacon of hope for many others.

"Heart healthy cookbook for all" is more than just a collection of recipes; it is an invitation to participate in a story of empowerment, resilience, and the joy of embracing a heart-healthy lifestyle. Each dish within these pages carries a piece of this narrative—a story of rejuvenation, flavor, and the art of savoring life with a healthy heart.

As you turn the pages of this cookbook, imagine joining Jane in her kitchen, where the aroma of nutritious ingredients mingles with the warmth of shared stories and the laughter that accompanies the creation of delicious meals.

Let these recipes be not just instructions but companions on your own unique journey toward heart-conscious living.

Welcome to Heart healthy cookbook for all, where the alchemy of flavors meets the poetry of heart wellness. May this cookbook inspire you to craft your own story of health, resilience, and the joyous celebration of a heart beating strong.

The Importance of Heart-Friendly Eating

In the symphony of our well-being, the heart stands as the conductor, orchestrating the rhythms that sustain life. The choices we make in the realm of nutrition play a pivotal role in harmonizing this intricate melody. "Heart healthy cookbook for all: Easy Delicious, Low Fat, Low Sodium Heart Healthy Recipes" is not just a cookbook; it is a guide that underscores the paramount importance of heart-friendly eating.

Our hearts, resilient and ceaselessly at work, deserve thoughtful care and consideration.

Heart-friendly eating is not a restrictive regimen but a celebration of nourishment that supports cardiovascular health. It is a lifestyle that embraces foods rich in nutrients, fiber, and antioxidants while minimizing the intake of saturated fats, cholesterol, and sodium.

The significance of heart-friendly eating extends beyond the prevention of cardiovascular diseases; it is a proactive approach to overall well-being. By making mindful choices in our daily meals, we contribute to maintaining healthy blood pressure, cholesterol levels, and weight. These, in turn, serve as pillars for a robust cardiovascular system, reducing the risk of heart-related ailments.

Embracing heart-friendly eating is not about sacrifice; it's about savoring the abundance of wholesome, flavorful foods that fortify our bodies. Fresh fruits and vegetables, whole grains, lean proteins, and heart-healthy fats become the building blocks of a diet that nurtures and sustains. The recipes within this cookbook are crafted with these principles in mind, offering a palette of delicious options that prioritize both health and taste.

Beyond the physical aspects, heart-friendly eating has a profound impact on our overall quality of life. Increased energy, improved mood, and enhanced cognitive function are among the many benefits that accompany a heart-conscious lifestyle. As we navigate the complexities of modern living, the choices we make at the dining table become a powerful tool for nurturing not only our bodies but also our hearts and minds.

In "Heart healthy cookbook for all," we invite you to embark on a journey where every meal is a conscious act of self-care. May the importance of heart-friendly eating resonate with you, inspiring a culinary adventure that transforms not just your diet but your entire approach to well-being.

FOUNDATIONS OF HEART-HEALTHY CUISINE

Understanding Heart Health

In the intricate tapestry of human physiology, the heart stands as a resilient maestro orchestrating the symphony of life. To embark on a journey of heart-friendly eating, it is essential to delve into the depths of understanding heart health – to recognize the nuances of this vital organ and the profound impact our lifestyle choices can have on its well-being.

- **The Heart's Unspoken Language**

Our hearts, tirelessly beating an average of 100,000 times a day, are eloquent storytellers of our overall health. Understanding their language involves deciphering the rhythms, interpreting the signals, and acknowledging the factors that contribute to their harmony or discord.

Heart health encompasses not only the absence of disease but the cultivation of a robust cardiovascular system that propels us toward vitality.

- **Risk Factors and Guardians of the Heart**

Heart health is a delicate balance influenced by both modifiable and non-modifiable factors.

Genetics, age, and gender play their roles, but lifestyle choices wield considerable influence. Smoking, sedentary living, excessive alcohol consumption, and a diet rich in saturated fats and sugars can tip the scales toward cardiovascular risks.

Conversely, adopting heart-friendly habits becomes the armor shielding the heart from potential threats. Regular physical activity, maintaining a healthy weight, managing stress, and, significantly, adopting a heart-conscious diet contribute to fortifying this protective shield.

- **The Cardiovascular Symphony: Blood Pressure, Cholesterol, and Beyond**

Within the intricacies of heart health, blood pressure and cholesterol levels emerge as key players in the cardiovascular symphony. Hypertension strains the heart, while elevated cholesterol levels contribute to arterial plaque formation. Unchecked, these factors can lead to conditions such as heart disease and stroke.

Understanding the roles of high-density lipoprotein (HDL), low-density lipoprotein (LDL), and triglycerides equips us with the knowledge needed to make informed dietary choices.

Crafting a heart-friendly diet involves not only embracing nutrient-rich foods but also moderating intake of saturated and trans fats, sodium, and refined sugars.

- **Listening to the Heart's Whispers: Early Warning Signs**

In the narrative of heart health, recognizing the subtle whispers of distress is crucial. Awareness of early warning signs, such as chest discomfort, shortness of breath, and fatigue, prompts timely action and can be instrumental in preventing further complications.

As we embark on the culinary journey of heart-friendly eating, understanding the language of the heart lays the foundation for informed choices. By appreciating the intricacies of heart health, we empower ourselves to make decisions that resonate with the well-being of this vital organ. In the upcoming chapters, we will translate this understanding into practical culinary wisdom, exploring recipes that nourish not only the body but also the symphony of our beating hearts.

Healthy Fats: Opting for heart-healthy fats, like those found in avocados, nuts, and olive oil, provides a source of monounsaturated and polyunsaturated fats that contribute to cardiovascular well-being.

- **Balancing Act: The Art of Portion Control**

Beyond the selection of nutrient-dense ingredients, mastering the art of portion control is a fundamental aspect of heart-healthy eating. While the quality of our food choices matters, so too does the quantity. Understanding appropriate serving sizes helps maintain a balance of essential nutrients while preventing overconsumption of calories.

- **Mindful Preparation: Cooking Techniques for Heart Wellness**

The way we prepare our meals can significantly impact their nutritional content. Adopting heart-conscious cooking techniques ensures that the integrity of our chosen ingredients is preserved, maximizing their health benefits.

Techniques such as grilling, baking, steaming, and sautéing with heart-healthy oils allow us to retain the nutritional value of our foods without excessive use of added fats and sodium.

As we embark on this culinary journey, let the foundations of heart-healthy cuisine serve as your compass, guiding you toward a path of nourishment, vitality, and the joy of savoring meals that not only tantalize the taste buds but also honor the well-being of your heart.

In the chapters to come, we'll delve deeper into these principles, exploring delicious recipes that embody the essence of heart-conscious living.

Key Nutrients for Cardiovascular Wellness

In the intricate dance of heart health, the spotlight falls on the protagonists—the key nutrients that choreograph the symphony of well-being within our cardiovascular system.

This chapter unveils the nutritional powerhouses essential for maintaining a resilient heart and explores how incorporating these elements into our diets can be a transformative act of self-care.

- **Omega-3 Fatty Acids: Guardians of Cardiovascular Harmony**

Like a gentle breeze through a meadow, omega-3 fatty acids bring a sense of tranquility to the cardiovascular landscape. Found abundantly in fatty fish such as salmon, mackerel, and walnuts, these essential fatty acids not only contribute to heart health but also wield anti-inflammatory properties. Their harmonious presence helps reduce the risk of heart disease by lowering blood pressure, improving cholesterol levels, and promoting overall vascular health.

- **Fiber: The Sustaining Thread of Cardiovascular Resilience**

Picture fiber as the weaver of cardiovascular resilience, intricately threading its way through our diets to fortify heart health. Abundant in fruits, vegetables, whole grains, and legumes, fiber contributes to a lower risk of heart disease by reducing cholesterol levels and supporting healthy blood pressure. Its role extends beyond cardiovascular benefits, embracing digestive health and satiety, making it a fundamental component of a heart-conscious diet.

- **Antioxidants: Nature's Protective Shields**

In the battle against oxidative stress, antioxidants emerge as nature's formidable protectors. Abundant in colorful fruits and vegetables, these compounds neutralize free radicals, preventing cellular damage and inflammation.

By incorporating a rainbow of antioxidants into our diets, we not only support cardiovascular health but also bolster our immune systems and promote overall well-being.

- **Potassium: The Electrolyte Maestro**

Potassium orchestrates the delicate balance of electrolytes, playing a crucial role in maintaining healthy blood pressure and supporting proper heart function. Found in bananas, oranges, potatoes, and leafy greens, potassium acts as a counterforce to sodium, helping regulate fluid balance and contributing to cardiovascular harmony.

- **Calcium and Magnesium: Bone and Heart Allies**

Beyond their role in bone health, calcium and magnesium form a dynamic duo that supports cardiovascular wellness.

Calcium contributes to blood clotting and muscle function, while magnesium helps regulate blood pressure and supports heart rhythm.

Dairy products, leafy greens, nuts, and seeds are rich sources of these essential minerals.

Understanding the roles of these key nutrients empowers us to craft meals that resonate with the well-being of our hearts. As we delve into heart-friendly recipes in the chapters to come, let these nutritional elements be our guiding lights, illuminating a path toward a robust and resilient cardiovascular symphony.

Tips for Heart-Conscious Cooking

Navigating the realm of heart-conscious cooking is a culinary journey that seamlessly blends flavor and well-being. This chapter serves as a guide, offering practical tips and creative insights to transform your time in the kitchen into a symphony of heart-friendly delights. Let these suggestions inspire your culinary prowess as you embark on crafting nourishing and delectable meals.

1. **Embrace Lean Proteins:** Opt for lean protein sources such as poultry, fish, tofu, and legumes. These choices provide essential amino acids without the excess saturated fats found in certain red meats. Experiment with flavorful marinades

and herbs to enhance the taste without compromising on health.

2. **Choose Heart-Healthy Fats:** Replace saturated and trans fats with heart-healthy fats such as those found in avocados, nuts, seeds, and olive oil. These fats contribute to lower cholesterol levels and support overall cardiovascular wellness. Incorporate them into salads, dressings, and cooking to add richness and flavor.

3. **Explore Whole Grains:** Swap refined grains for whole grains like quinoa, brown rice, and oats. Whole grains are rich in fiber, which aids in managing cholesterol levels and promoting heart health.

   Explore a variety of grains to add texture and depth to your dishes.

4. **Prioritize Plant-Based Options:** Integrate more plant-based meals into your repertoire. Explore the world of colorful vegetables, fruits, and legumes to create vibrant, nutrient-packed dishes. Plant-based diets are associated with lower risks of heart disease and offer a diverse range of flavors and textures.

5. **Mindful Portion Control:** Practice mindful eating by paying attention to portion sizes.

Be conscious of serving sizes to avoid overeating and promote a balanced intake of nutrients. Savor each bite and allow yourself to enjoy the flavors without feeling rushed.

6. **Reduce Sodium Intake:** Be mindful of sodium content in your recipes. Opt for herbs, spices, and other flavor enhancers to season your dishes instead of relying heavily on salt.
Lowering sodium intake contributes to better blood pressure management and heart health.

7. **Get Creative with Cooking Techniques:** Experiment with heart-friendly cooking methods such as grilling, baking, steaming, and sautéing. These techniques retain the nutritional value of ingredients without excessive use of added fats. Explore the world of culinary creativity while preserving the health benefits of your chosen ingredients.

8. **Hydration with a Twist:** Stay hydrated with heart-healthy beverages like herbal teas and infused water. Limit sugary drinks and excessive caffeine intake. Proper hydration supports overall health and can be a delightful addition to your heart-conscious lifestyle.

9. **Choose Natural Sweeteners:** Opt for natural sweeteners like honey, maple syrup, or agave nectar instead of refined sugars. These alternatives add sweetness to your recipes

while providing some additional nutrients and a gentler impact on blood sugar levels.

10. **Listen to Your Body:** Pay attention to how your body responds to different foods. Everyone's nutritional needs are unique, so tailor your diet to what makes you feel best. Consult with healthcare

11. **Smoothie** professionals or nutritionists to create a personalized and sustainable heart-conscious eating plan.

By incorporating these tips into your culinary repertoire, you'll embark on a flavorful and heart-conscious journey, savoring the joys of nourishing your body while cultivating a love for heart-friendly cooking.

BREAKFAST BOOSTERS

Energizing Morning Smoothies

As the sun rises, bringing with it the promise of a new day, there's no better way to kickstart your morning than with a vibrant and nutrient-packed smoothie. This chapter unfolds a symphony of flavors and vitality, offering a collection of energizing morning smoothies designed to nourish your body, awaken your senses, and set a positive tone for the day ahead.

1. Sunrise Citrus Burst:

Ingredients: Oranges, Pineapple, Greek Yogurt, Chia Seeds

Instructions:

- Peel and segment the oranges.
- Chop the pineapple into chunks.
- In a blender, combine the oranges, pineapple, Greek yogurt, and chia seeds.
- Blend until smooth and creamy.
- Pour into a glass and garnish with a sprinkle of chia seeds.

2. Berry Bliss Awakening:

Ingredients: Mixed Berries (Strawberries, Blueberries, Raspberries), Banana, Almond Milk, Spinach

Instructions:

- Wash and hull the berries.
- Peel and slice the banana.
- In a blender, combine the mixed berries, banana, almond milk, and spinach.
- Blend until smooth.
- Pour into a glass and enjoy the burst of berry freshness.

3. Green Goddess Power:

Ingredients: Kale, Cucumber, Green Apple, Avocado, Coconut Water

Instructions:

- Destem the kale leaves.
- Dice the cucumber, green apple, and avocado.
- In a blender, combine the kale, cucumber, green apple, avocado, and coconut water.
- Blend until silky smooth.
- Pour into a glass and savor the green goodness.

4. Tropical Turmeric Delight:

Ingredients: Mango, Pineapple, Turmeric, Coconut Milk, Ginger

Instructions:

- Peel and cube the mango and pineapple.

- Peel and grate the turmeric and ginger.
- In a blender, combine the mango, pineapple, turmeric, coconut milk, and ginger.
- Blend until the mixture is velvety.
- Pour into a glass and relish the tropical flavors.

5. Protein-Packed Peanut Butter Banana Boost:

Ingredients: Banana, Peanut Butter, Greek Yogurt, Almond Milk, Protein Powder

Instructions:

- Peel and slice the banana.
- In a blender, combine the banana, peanut butter, Greek yogurt, almond milk, and protein powder.
- Blend until creamy.
- Pour into a glass and sprinkle with a pinch of protein powder if desired.

Note: Adjust the consistency by adding more almond milk if needed.

6. Energizing Espresso Smoothie:

Ingredients: Cold Brew Coffee, Banana, Almond Butter, Dates, Almond Milk

Instructions:

- Brew cold brew coffee or use pre-made cold brew.
- Peel and slice the banana.
- In a blender, combine the cold brew coffee, banana, almond butter, dates, and almond milk.
- Blend until smooth and frothy.
- Pour into a glass and savor the coffee-infused energy.

7. Oatmeal Cookie Morning Bliss:

Ingredients: Rolled Oats, Banana, Cinnamon, Almond Milk, Vanilla Extract

Instructions:

- Peel and slice the banana.
- In a blender, combine the rolled oats, banana, cinnamon, almond milk, and vanilla extract.
- Blend until the oats are finely ground.
- Pour into a glass and enjoy the nostalgic oatmeal cookie flavor.

8. Avocado Mango Tango:

Ingredients: Avocado, Mango, Lime Juice, Spinach, Coconut Water

Instructions:

- Peel and dice the avocado and mango.

- In a blender, combine the avocado, mango, lime juice, spinach, and coconut water.
- Blend until silky and smooth.
- Pour into a glass and revel in the tropical tango.

9. Blueberry Almond Bliss:

Ingredients: Blueberries, Almonds, Banana, Greek Yogurt, Almond Milk

Instructions:

- Wash the blueberries.
- Peel and slice the banana.
- In a blender, combine the blueberries, almonds, banana, Greek yogurt, and almond milk.
- Blend until creamy.
- Pour into a glass and enjoy the blueberry-almond fusion.

10. Chia Cherry Refresher:

Ingredients: Cherries, Chia Seeds, Coconut Water, Lime Zest, Honey

Instructions:

- Pit and halve the cherries.

- In a blender, combine the cherries, chia seeds, coconut water, lime zest, and honey.
- Blend until the chia seeds are evenly distributed.
- Pour into a glass and relish the refreshing chia-cherry goodness.

Note: Allow chia seeds to soak for a few minutes before consuming for a thicker consistency.

Nutrient-Packed Oatmeal Variations

Elevate your breakfast routine with a symphony of nutrient-packed oatmeal variations that not only tantalize your taste buds but also provide a wholesome start to your day. From classic combinations to inventive twists, these recipes showcase the versatility of oats, ensuring a satisfying and nutritious morning meal.

1. Classic Maple Pecan Oatmeal:

Ingredients:

- 1 cup Rolled Oats
- 2 tablespoons Maple Syrup
- 2 tablespoons Chopped Pecans
- 1/2 teaspoon Cinnamon

Instructions:

- Cook rolled oats according to package instructions.
- Drizzle with maple syrup.
- Sprinkle with chopped pecans and a dash of cinnamon.
- Stir and enjoy the classic warmth of maple and pecans.

2. Berry Nut Bliss Oatmeal:

Ingredients:

- 1 cup Steel-Cut Oats
- 1 cup Mixed Berries (Strawberries, Blueberries, Raspberries)
- 2 tablespoons Almonds, sliced
- 1 tablespoon Honey

Instructions:

- Cook steel-cut oats with water or milk.
- Top with a medley of fresh berries.
- Garnish with sliced almonds.
- Drizzle with honey for a delightful burst of flavors.

3. Apple Cinnamon Crunch Oatmeal:

Ingredients:

- 1 cup Old-Fashioned Oats
- 1 cup Diced Apples
- 2 tablespoons Chopped Walnuts
- 1/2 teaspoon Ground Cinnamon

Instructions:

- Cook old-fashioned oats until creamy.
- Add diced apples and stir until softened.

- Top with chopped walnuts and a generous sprinkle of ground cinnamon.
- Dive into the comforting embrace of apple and cinnamon.

4. Tropical Coconut Oatmeal:

Ingredients:

- 1 cup Rolled Oats
- 1 cup Fresh Pineapple Chunks
- 2 tablespoons Shredded Coconut
- 1 tablespoon Chia Seeds

Instructions:

- Cook rolled oats with coconut milk.
- Stir in fresh pineapple chunks.
- Sprinkle with shredded coconut and chia seeds.
- Transport yourself to a tropical paradise with each spoonful.

5. Peanut Butter Banana Crunch Oatmeal:

Ingredients:

- 1 cup Quick Oats
- 1 Banana, sliced
- 2 tablespoons Peanut Butter
- Granola for topping

Instructions:

- Prepare quick oats according to package instructions.

- Top with sliced bananas.

- Drizzle with a dollop of peanut butter.

- Finish with a crunchy layer of granola for added texture.

6. Chocolate Almond Joy Oatmeal:

Ingredients:

- 1 cup Steel-Cut Oats

- 1 tablespoon Cocoa Powder

- 2 tablespoons Sliced Almonds

- 2 tablespoons Coconut Flakes

Instructions:

- Cook steel-cut oats with a dash of cocoa powder.

- Garnish with sliced almonds and coconut flakes.

- Indulge in the heavenly combination of chocolate and almonds.

7. Savory Spinach and Feta Oatmeal:

Ingredients:

- 1 cup Old-Fashioned Oats

- 1 cup Fresh Spinach

- 2 tablespoons Feta Cheese, crumbled

- Cherry Tomatoes, halved

Instructions:

- Cook old-fashioned oats with water or broth.

- Stir in fresh spinach until wilted.

- Top with crumbled feta cheese and halved cherry tomatoes.

- Experience a savory twist on oatmeal with this delightful combination.

8. Maple Pumpkin Pie Oatmeal:

Ingredients:

- 1 cup Rolled Oats

- 1/2 cup Pumpkin Puree

- 2 tablespoons Maple Syrup

- Pumpkin Spice Blend to taste

Instructions:

- Cook rolled oats with water or milk.

- Stir in pumpkin puree and a drizzle of maple syrup.

- Sprinkle with a pumpkin spice blend for a taste of autumn in a bowl.

9. Mediterranean-Inspired Oat Bowl:

Ingredients:

- 1 cup Steel-Cut Oats

- Kalamata Olives, sliced

- Cherry Tomatoes, halved

- 2 tablespoons Feta Cheese, crumbled

- Olive Oil for drizzling

Instructions:

- Cook steel-cut oats with water or broth.

- Top with sliced Kalamata olives, halved cherry tomatoes, and crumbled feta cheese.

- Drizzle with olive oil for a savory and satisfying breakfast.

10. Blueberry Lemon Poppy Seed Oatmeal:

Ingredients:

- 1 cup Quick Oats

- 1 cup Fresh Blueberries

- Lemon Zest to taste

- Poppy Seeds for sprinkling

Instructions:

- Prepare quick oats according to package instructions.

- Stir in fresh blueberries and lemon zest.

- Sprinkle with poppy seeds for a burst of citrusy goodness.

Experiment with these nutrient-packed oatmeal variations to discover your favorite morning bowl. Whether you prefer sweet or savory, there's an oatmeal creation to suit every palate and provide a nourishing start to your day.

Heart-Healthy Breakfast Bites

Start your day on a heart-healthy note with these delectable and nutritious breakfast bites. Packed with wholesome ingredients and bursting with flavor, these recipes are designed to fuel your morning and support cardiovascular well-being. From grab-and-go options to leisurely breakfast delights, these bites are a delightful addition to your heart-conscious lifestyle.

1. Quinoa Breakfast Muffins:

Ingredients:

- 1 cup Cooked Quinoa
- 1/2 cup Spinach, finely chopped
- 1/4 cup Feta Cheese, crumbled
- 2 Eggs
- Salt and Pepper to taste

Instructions:

- Preheat oven to 350°F (175°C).
- In a bowl, mix cooked quinoa, chopped spinach, feta cheese, eggs, salt, and pepper.
- Spoon the mixture into muffin cups.
- Bake for 20-25 minutes or until set.
- Allow to cool slightly before serving.

2. Berry-Almond Chia Pudding Cups:

Ingredients:

- 1/4 cup Chia Seeds
- 1 cup Almond Milk
- Mixed Berries (Strawberries, Blueberries, Raspberries)
- Almonds, sliced

Instructions:

- In a jar, mix chia seeds and almond milk. Refrigerate overnight.
- Layer chia pudding with mixed berries in small cups.
- Top with sliced almonds before serving.

3. Sweet Potato Breakfast Bites:

Ingredients:

- 1 cup Sweet Potato, grated
- 2 Eggs
- 1/4 cup Whole Wheat Flour
- 1/2 teaspoon Baking Powder
- Cinnamon to taste

Instructions:

- Preheat oven to 375°F (190°C).
- In a bowl, combine grated sweet potato, eggs, whole wheat flour, baking powder, and cinnamon.
- Spoon the mixture into a mini muffin tin.
- Bake for 15-18 minutes or until golden brown.

4. Greek Yogurt Parfait Bites:

Ingredients:

- Greek Yogurt
- Granola
- Mixed Berries
- Honey for drizzling

Instructions:

- In mini cups, layer Greek yogurt, granola, and mixed berries.
- Drizzle with honey before serving.
- Spinach and Feta Egg Cups.

Ingredients:

- Eggs
- Spinach, chopped
- Feta Cheese, crumbled
- Salt and Pepper to taste

Instructions:

- Preheat oven to 375°F (190°C).
- In a muffin tin, place chopped spinach and crumbled feta.
- Crack an egg into each cup.
- Season with salt and pepper.
- Bake for 12-15 minutes or until the eggs are set.

6. Oatmeal Banana Bites:

Ingredients:

- 1 cup Old-Fashioned Oats
- 2 Bananas, mashed
- 1/4 cup Almond Butter
- Cinnamon to taste

Instructions:

- Preheat oven to 350°F (175°C).
- In a bowl, mix oats, mashed bananas, almond butter, and cinnamon.
- Drop spoonful onto a baking sheet.
- Bake for 10-12 minutes or until golden brown.

7. Avocado and Tomato Toast Bites:

Ingredients:

- Whole Grain Bread, toasted and cut into bite-sized pieces
- Avocado, mashed
- Cherry Tomatoes, sliced
- Sea Salt and Black Pepper to taste

Instructions:

- Spread mashed avocado on toasted bread pieces.
- Top with sliced cherry tomatoes.
- Season with sea salt and black pepper.

8. Blueberry Chia Breakfast Bars:

Ingredients:

- 1 cup Rolled Oats
- 1/4 cup Chia Seeds
- 1/2 cup Blueberries
- 1/4 cup Almond Butter
- 1/4 cup Honey

Instructions:

- Mix rolled oats, chia seeds, blueberries, almond butter, and honey in a bowl.
- Press the mixture into a lined baking dish.
- Refrigerate for at least 2 hours before cutting into bars.

9. Almond and Apricot Energy Bites:

Ingredients:

- Almonds
- Dried Apricots
- Honey
- Flaxseeds

Instructions:

- In a food processor, blend almonds, dried apricots, honey, and flaxseeds until a sticky mixture forms.
- Roll into bite-sized balls and refrigerate for firmness.

10. Veggie Breakfast Skewers:

Ingredients:

- Cherry Tomatoes
- Cucumber, sliced
- Mozzarella Balls
- Basil Leaves

Instructions:

- Thread cherry tomatoes, cucumber slices, mozzarella balls, and basil leaves onto skewers.
- Arrange on a plate for a colorful and refreshing breakfast.

These heart-healthy breakfast bites offer a delightful array of flavors and textures, ensuring a nourishing and satisfying start to your day. Whether you're in a rush or have time to savor, these recipes cater to a heart-conscious lifestyle with every delicious bite.

WHOLESOME SOUPS AND SALADS

Hearty Lentil Soup Recipe

Warm, comforting, and rich in nutrients, this hearty lentil soup is a wholesome dish that nourishes both body and soul. Packed with protein, fiber, and an array of aromatic spices, it's a perfect addition to your collection of heart-healthy recipes.

Ingredients:

- 1 cup dry Brown Lentils, rinsed and drained
- 1 large Onion, diced
- 2 Carrots, diced
- 2 Celery stalks, diced
- 3 cloves Garlic, minced
- 1 can (14 oz) Diced Tomatoes, undrained
- 6 cups Vegetable Broth
- 1 teaspoon Ground Cumin
- 1 teaspoon Ground Coriander
- 1/2 teaspoon Smoked Paprika
- 1/2 teaspoon Turmeric
- 1/2 teaspoon Chili Powder (adjust to taste)
- Salt and Pepper to taste
- 2 tablespoons Olive Oil
- Fresh Parsley for garnish (optional)

- Lemon wedges for serving (optional)

Instructions:

1. Prepare Lentils

- Rinse the lentils under cold water and drain.

2. Sauté Vegetables

- In a large soup pot, heat olive oil over medium heat.
- Add diced onions, carrots, and celery. Sauté until vegetables are softened, about 5-7 minutes.

3. Add Aromatics

- Stir in minced garlic and continue to sauté for another minute until fragrant.

4. Spice it Up

- Add ground cumin, ground coriander, smoked paprika, turmeric, and chili powder to the vegetables.
- Stir well to coat the vegetables in the spices.

5. Combine Lentils and Broth

- Add the rinsed lentils to the pot and pour in the vegetable broth.
- Include the undrained diced tomatoes.

6. Season and Simmer

- Season the soup with salt and pepper to taste.
- Bring the soup to a boil, then reduce the heat to low, cover, and let it simmer for about 25-30 minutes or until lentils are tender.

7. Adjust Consistency

- If the soup is too thick, you can add more vegetable broth until you reach your desired consistency.

8. Taste and Adjust

- Taste the soup and adjust the seasonings according to your preferences. You might want to add a bit more salt, pepper, or spices.

9. Serve

- Ladle the soup into bowls.
- Garnish with fresh parsley if desired.
- Serve with lemon wedges on the side for a burst of citrus flavor.
- Enjoy this hearty lentil soup on its own or with a slice of whole-grain bread for a complete and satisfying meal.

Note: Feel free to customize this recipe by adding other vegetables like spinach, kale, or zucchini. You can also experiment with different herbs and spices to suit your taste preferences.

Spinach and Walnut Salad with Citrus Vinaigrette Recipe

Create a refreshing and nutritious spinach and walnut salad with a zesty citrus vinaigrette. This vibrant dish is not only packed with essential nutrients but also delights the palate with a perfect balance of flavors.

Ingredients:

For the Salad:

- 6 cups Fresh Spinach leaves, washed and dried
- 1 cup Cherry Tomatoes, halved
- 1/2 cup Red Onion, thinly sliced
- 1/2 cup Walnuts, toasted
- 1/4 cup Feta Cheese, crumbled (optional)
- Salt and Pepper to taste

For the Citrus Vinaigrette:

- 1/4 cup Olive Oil
- 2 tablespoons Fresh Orange Juice
- 1 tablespoon Fresh Lemon Juice

- 1 teaspoon Honey
- 1 teaspoon Dijon Mustard
- 1 clove Garlic, minced
- Salt and Pepper to taste

Instructions:

1. Prepare the Citrus Vinaigrette:

- In a small bowl, whisk together olive oil, fresh orange juice, fresh lemon juice, honey, Dijon mustard, minced garlic, salt, and pepper. Set aside.

2. Toast the Walnuts:

- In a dry skillet over medium heat, toast the walnuts until they become fragrant, stirring frequently. Be careful not to burn them. Remove from heat and let them cool.

3. Assemble the Salad:

- In a large salad bowl, combine the fresh spinach leaves, halved cherry tomatoes, thinly sliced red onion, and toasted walnuts.

4. Add Optional Feta Cheese:

- If using feta cheese, crumble it over the salad.

5. Drizzle with Citrus Vinaigrette:

- Drizzle the citrus vinaigrette over the salad. Start with a portion and add more as needed, tossing the salad gently to coat the ingredients evenly.

6. Season to Taste:

- Season the salad with salt and pepper to taste. Toss again to combine.

7. Serve Immediately:

- Serve the spinach and walnut salad immediately, ensuring the vibrant flavors are at their peak.

8. Optional Garnish:

- For an extra burst of citrus flavor, you can garnish the salad with a bit of grated orange or lemon zest.

9. Enjoy:

- Enjoy this refreshing and nutrient-packed salad as a light and satisfying meal on its own or as a delightful side dish.

Note: Feel free to customize the salad by adding ingredients like sliced strawberries, avocado, or grilled chicken for additional flavor and texture variations. Adjust the quantity of the vinaigrette according to your taste preferences.

Quinoa and Vegetable Power Bowl Recipe

Fuel your day with a nutrient-packed quinoa and vegetable power bowl. This wholesome and satisfying dish combines the goodness of quinoa with a variety of colorful vegetables, creating a vibrant and delicious meal that supports your well-being.

Ingredients:

For the Quinoa:

- 1 cup Quinoa, rinsed
- 2 cups Vegetable Broth or Water
- 1/2 teaspoon Olive Oil
- Salt to taste

For the Vegetable Medley:

- 1 tablespoon Olive Oil
- 1 Red Bell Pepper, diced
- 1 Yellow Bell Pepper, diced
- 1 Zucchini, diced
- 1 Carrot, julienned
- 1 cup Cherry Tomatoes, halved
- 2 cups Baby Spinach, washed
- 2 cloves Garlic, minced
- Salt and Pepper to taste
- 1 teaspoon Dried Italian Herbs (optional)

For the Lemon-Tahini Dressing:

- 3 tablespoons Tahini

- 2 tablespoons Fresh Lemon Juice

- 2 tablespoons Water

- 1 clove Garlic, minced

- Salt and Pepper to taste

Optional Toppings:

- Avocado slices

- Pumpkin seeds

- Feta cheese (optional)

Instructions:

1. Prepare Quinoa:

- In a saucepan, combine quinoa, vegetable broth or water, olive oil, and a pinch of salt.

Bring to a boil, then reduce heat, cover, and simmer for 15-20 minutes or until quinoa is cooked and water is absorbed. Fluff with a fork and set aside.

2. Make Lemon-Tahini Dressing:

- In a small bowl, whisk together tahini, fresh lemon juice, water, minced garlic, salt, and pepper. Adjust the consistency by adding more water if needed. Set aside.

3. Sauté Vegetables:

- In a large skillet, heat olive oil over medium heat.
- Add diced red and yellow bell peppers, zucchini, julienned carrot, and minced garlic.
- Sauté for 5-7 minutes or until the vegetables are tender yet still vibrant.

4. Add Cherry Tomatoes and Spinach:

- Add cherry tomatoes to the skillet and sauté for an additional 2-3 minutes until they soften.
- Stir in baby spinach and cook until wilted.

5. Season and Add Quinoa:

- Season the vegetable medley with salt, pepper, and dried Italian herbs if using.
- Add the cooked quinoa to the skillet and toss everything together until well combined. Adjust seasoning if necessary.

6. Assemble the Power Bowl:

- Divide the quinoa and vegetable mixture into serving bowls.

7. Drizzle with Lemon-Tahini Dressing:

- Drizzle the lemon-tahini dressing over each power bowl.

8. Optional Toppings:

- Garnish with avocado slices, pumpkin seeds, and feta cheese if desired.

9. Serve:

Serve the quinoa and vegetable power bowl immediately, allowing everyone to customize their bowls with additional toppings.

Enjoy this vibrant and nutrient-rich power bowl as a complete and nourishing meal. Feel free to customize this recipe by adding your favorite vegetables or protein sources like grilled chicken, chickpeas, or tofu. Adjust the dressing ingredients to suit your taste preferences.

LEAN PROTEIN DELIGHTS

Baked Salmon with Lemon-Dill Sauce Recipe

Elevate your dinner with this simple yet elegant baked salmon dish. The combination of flaky salmon with a zesty lemon-dill sauce creates a delightful harmony of flavors. This recipe is not only delicious but also a healthy choice for a heart-conscious meal.

Ingredients:

For the Baked Salmon:

- 4 Salmon Fillets
- 2 tablespoons Olive Oil
- Salt and Pepper to taste
- Lemon Slices for garnish

For the Lemon-Dill Sauce:

- 1/2 cup Greek Yogurt
- 2 tablespoons Fresh Dill, finely chopped
- 1 tablespoon Dijon Mustard
- 1 tablespoon Fresh Lemon Juice
- 1 clove Garlic, minced
- Salt and Pepper to taste

Instructions:

1. Preheat the Oven:

- Preheat your oven to 400°F (200°C).

2. Prepare the Salmon:

- Pat the salmon fillets dry with a paper towel.
- Place the salmon fillets on a baking sheet lined with parchment paper.

3. Season the Salmon:

- Drizzle olive oil over the salmon fillets, ensuring they are well-coated.
- Season with salt and pepper to taste.

4. Bake the Salmon:

- Bake the salmon in the preheated oven for 12-15 minutes or until the salmon flakes easily with a fork.

5. Prepare the Lemon-Dill Sauce:

- While the salmon is baking, prepare the lemon-dill sauce.
- In a bowl, mix together Greek yogurt, finely chopped fresh dill, Dijon mustard, fresh lemon juice, minced garlic, salt, and pepper.

6. Check Salmon for Doneness:

- Remove the salmon from the oven and check for doneness. The salmon should be opaque and easily flaked with a fork.

7. Serve with Lemon-Dill Sauce:

- Plate the baked salmon fillets.
- Drizzle each fillet with the prepared lemon-dill sauce.

8. Garnish and Serve:

- Garnish the salmon with lemon slices for a fresh touch.
- Serve immediately, and enjoy the succulent baked salmon with the flavorful lemon-dill sauce.

Note:

- You can adjust the baking time based on the thickness of your salmon fillets. Thicker fillets may require a few additional minutes in the oven.
- Experiment with additional herbs or spices in the lemon-dill sauce to suit your taste preferences.
- This dish pairs well with steamed vegetables, quinoa, or a light salad for a well-rounded meal.

Grilled Chicken and Avocado Quinoa Bowl Recipe

Create a wholesome and satisfying meal with this grilled chicken and avocado quinoa bowl. Packed with protein, fiber, and healthy fats, this dish not only tastes delicious but also provides a nourishing combination for a heart-healthy lifestyle.

Ingredients:

For the Grilled Chicken:

- 2 Chicken Breasts, boneless and skinless
- 2 tablespoons Olive Oil
- 1 teaspoon Paprika
- 1 teaspoon Garlic Powder
- 1 teaspoon Dried Oregano
- Salt and Pepper to taste
- Lemon wedges for serving

For the Quinoa:

- 1 cup Quinoa, rinsed
- 2 cups Chicken Broth or Water
- Salt to taste

For the Avocado Salsa:

- 2 Avocados, diced
- 1 cup Cherry Tomatoes, halved
- 1/4 cup Red Onion, finely chopped
- 1/4 cup Fresh Cilantro, chopped
- 1 Lime, juiced
- Salt and Pepper to taste

Optional Garnish:

- Greek Yogurt or Sour Cream
- Feta Cheese, crumbled

Instructions:

1. Marinate and Grill the Chicken:

- In a bowl, combine olive oil, paprika, garlic powder, dried oregano, salt, and pepper.
- Coat the chicken breasts with the marinade and let them marinate for at least 30 minutes.
- Preheat the grill or grill pan over medium-high heat.
- Grill the chicken breasts for about 6-8 minutes per side or until fully cooked.
- Squeeze fresh lemon juice over the grilled chicken before slicing.

2. Prepare Quinoa:

- In a saucepan, combine quinoa, chicken broth or water, and salt.

- Bring to a boil, then reduce heat, cover, and simmer for 15-20 minutes or until quinoa is cooked and liquid is absorbed.

- Fluff with a fork and set aside.

3. Make Avocado Salsa:

- In a bowl, combine diced avocados, halved cherry tomatoes, finely chopped red onion, chopped cilantro, lime juice, salt, and pepper. Toss gently to combine.

4. Assemble the Quinoa Bowl:

- Divide the cooked quinoa among serving bowls.

5. Add Grilled Chicken:

- Slice the grilled chicken breasts and arrange them on top of the quinoa.

6. Top with Avocado Salsa:

- Spoon the avocado salsa generously over the grilled chicken.

7. Optional Garnish:

- If desired, add a dollop of Greek yogurt or sour cream on the side of the bowl.

- Sprinkle crumbled feta cheese on top for an extra burst of flavor.

8. Serve and Enjoy:

- Serve the grilled chicken and avocado quinoa bowl immediately, offering additional lime wedges for squeezing over the dish.

Note:

- Customize the bowl with additional vegetables like roasted bell peppers, cucumbers, or black beans for added nutrition and flavor.

- Adjust the level of spice by adding chili powder or red pepper flakes to the grilled chicken marinade or avocado salsa.

- This bowl is versatile, making it an excellent choice for meal prep or a quick and nutritious dinner.

Vegetarian Protein-Packed Stir-Fry Recipe

Whip up a nutritious and protein-packed vegetarian stir-fry that's bursting with flavor and colorful vegetables. This quick and easy recipe is not only delicious but also a fantastic way to incorporate plant-based protein into your diet.

Ingredients:

For the Stir-Fry:

- 1 cup Firm Tofu, pressed and cubed
- 1 cup Tempeh, cubed
- 2 tablespoons Soy Sauce
- 1 tablespoon Sesame Oil
- 1 tablespoon Olive Oil
- 3 cloves Garlic, minced
- 1 tablespoon Ginger, minced
- 1 Red Bell Pepper, sliced
- 1 Yellow Bell Pepper, sliced
- 1 cup Broccoli Florets
- 1 Carrot, julienned
- 1 cup Snap Peas, trimmed
- 1 cup Cabbage, thinly sliced
- 1 cup Mushrooms, sliced
- 1/4 cup Green Onions, chopped (for garnish)
- Sesame Seeds (for garnish, optional)

For the Sauce:

- 3 tablespoons Soy Sauce
- 2 tablespoons Hoisin Sauce
- 1 tablespoon Rice Vinegar

- 1 tablespoon Maple Syrup or Agave Nectar
- 1 teaspoon Cornstarch mixed with 2 tablespoons water (for thickening)

Instructions:

1. Prepare Tofu and Tempeh:

- Press the tofu to remove excess water, then cube it.
- Cube the tempeh as well.
- In a bowl, marinate tofu and tempeh in soy sauce and sesame oil. Let them soak up the flavors for at least 15 minutes.

2. Make the Sauce:

- In a small bowl, whisk together soy sauce, hoisin sauce, rice vinegar, and maple syrup.
- In a separate small bowl, dissolve cornstarch in water to create a slurry for thickening the sauce.

3. Stir-Fry Tofu and Tempeh:

- Heat olive oil in a large wok or skillet over medium-high heat.
- Add marinated tofu and tempeh cubes. Stir-fry until they are golden brown and crispy on the edges.

4. Add Aromatics and Vegetables:

- Push the tofu and tempeh to one side of the wok, and add minced garlic and ginger to the other side. Sauté for about 30 seconds until fragrant.
- Add sliced bell peppers, broccoli, julienned carrot, snap peas, cabbage, and mushrooms. Stir-fry for 3-5 minutes until vegetables are slightly tender yet still crisp.

5. Combine and Sauce:

- Combine the tofu and tempeh with the vegetables in the wok.
- Pour the prepared sauce over the stir-fry. Toss everything together to coat evenly.

6. Thicken the Sauce:

- Drizzle the cornstarch slurry over the stir-fry and continue tossing until the sauce thickens.

7. Garnish and Serve:

- Garnish with chopped green onions and sesame seeds if desired.
- Serve the vegetarian protein-packed stir-fry over cooked brown rice or quinoa.

- Enjoy this delicious and protein-rich vegetarian stir-fry as a wholesome and satisfying meal.

Note:

- Feel free to customize the stir-fry with your favorite vegetables or add tofu and tempeh variations for more texture.
- Adjust the level of sweetness or saltiness in the sauce according to your taste preferences.
- Experiment with different stir-fry sauces or add a dash of sriracha for a spicy kick.

Plant-Powered Main Courses

Roasted Vegetable Lasagna Recipe

Indulge in a comforting and flavorful roasted vegetable lasagna that's both hearty and wholesome. Packed with layers of roasted vegetables, rich marinara sauce, and creamy béchamel, this vegetarian lasagna is a delightful twist on the classic favorite.

Ingredients:

For the Roasted Vegetables:

- 2 Zucchini, sliced
- 1 Eggplant, sliced
- 1 Red Bell Pepper, sliced
- 1 Yellow Bell Pepper, sliced
- 1 Red Onion, sliced
- 3 tablespoons Olive Oil
- Salt and Pepper to taste
- 2 teaspoons Italian Seasoning

For the Lasagna Layers:

- 9 Lasagna Noodles, cooked according to package instructions
- 2 cups Shredded Mozzarella Cheese
- 1 cup Grated Parmesan Cheese

- Fresh Basil leaves for garnish (optional)

For the Marinara Sauce:

- 2 cans (28 oz each) Crushed Tomatoes
- 3 cloves Garlic, minced
- 1 teaspoon Dried Oregano
- 1 teaspoon Dried Basil
- Salt and Pepper to taste
- 2 tablespoons Olive Oil

For the Béchamel Sauce:

- 1/4 cup Unsalted Butter
- 1/4 cup All-Purpose Flour
- 3 cups Milk
- Salt and Nutmeg to taste

Instructions:

1. Preheat the Oven:

- Preheat the oven to 400°F (200°C).

2. Roast the Vegetables:

- Toss sliced zucchini, eggplant, red bell pepper, yellow bell pepper, and red onion with olive oil, salt, pepper, and Italian seasoning.
- Spread the vegetables on a baking sheet and roast in the preheated oven for 20-25 minutes or until they are tender and slightly caramelized.

3. Prepare the Marinara Sauce:

- In a saucepan, heat olive oil over medium heat.
- Add minced garlic and sauté until fragrant.
- Pour in crushed tomatoes, dried oregano, dried basil, salt, and pepper.
- Simmer for 15-20 minutes, stirring occasionally.

4. Cook the Lasagna Noodles:

- Cook lasagna noodles according to package instructions. Drain and set aside.

5. Make the Béchamel Sauce:

- In a separate saucepan, melt butter over medium heat.
- Whisk in flour to create a roux.
- Gradually whisk in milk until smooth.
- Continue whisking until the sauce thickens.

- Season with salt and a pinch of nutmeg.

6. Assemble the Lasagna:

- In a greased baking dish, start layering with a thin coat of marinara sauce.
- Place a layer of cooked lasagna noodles on top.
- Spread a portion of roasted vegetables over the noodles.
- Drizzle with béchamel sauce and sprinkle with a combination of mozzarella and Parmesan cheese.
- Repeat the layers until the dish is filled, finishing with a layer of marinara sauce and a generous sprinkle of cheese on top.

7. Bake:

- Cover the baking dish with foil and bake in the preheated oven for 25-30 minutes.
- Uncover and bake for an additional 10-15 minutes or until the cheese is melted and bubbly.

8. Let it Rest:

- Allow the lasagna to rest for 10-15 minutes before slicing.

9. Garnish and Serve:

- Garnish with fresh basil leaves if desired.
- Serve the roasted vegetable lasagna warm, and enjoy the layers of flavors and textures.

Note:

- Feel free to add ricotta cheese or spinach between the layers for additional richness and nutritional value.
- Customize the vegetables according to your preferences or seasonal availability.
- This lasagna can be prepared ahead of time and refrigerated until ready to bake. Adjust baking time accordingly if starting from a chilled state.

Black Bean and Sweet Potato Chili Recipe

Warm up with a hearty and nutritious bowl of black bean and sweet potato chili. This flavorful vegetarian dish is not only satisfying but also packed with protein and fiber. Perfect for chilly days, this chili is a wholesome and comforting option for a heart-conscious meal.

Ingredients:

- 2 Sweet Potatoes, peeled and diced
- 2 cans (15 oz each) Black Beans, drained and rinsed
- 1 can (14 oz) Diced Tomatoes (with juices)
- 1 Red Bell Pepper, diced
- 1 Yellow Onion, diced
- 3 cloves Garlic, minced
- 1 Jalapeño, seeded and minced (optional, for heat)
- 1 cup Corn Kernels (fresh or frozen)

- 3 cups Vegetable Broth

- 2 tablespoons Chili Powder

- 1 tablespoon Ground Cumin

- 1 teaspoon Smoked Paprika

- 1 teaspoon Dried Oregano

- Salt and Pepper to taste

- 2 tablespoons Olive Oil

- Fresh Cilantro, chopped (for garnish)

- Avocado slices (for garnish, optional)

- Lime wedges (for serving)

Instructions:

1.Prepare Sweet Potatoes:

- Peel and dice the sweet potatoes into bite-sized cubes.

2. Sauté Vegetables:

- In a large pot, heat olive oil over medium heat.
- Add diced onions, minced garlic, and jalapeño (if using). Sauté until the onions are translucent.

3. Add Sweet Potatoes and Spices:

- Add diced sweet potatoes to the pot and stir well.

- Sprinkle chili powder, ground cumin, smoked paprika, dried oregano, salt, and pepper. Mix until the sweet potatoes are coated with the spices.

4. Combine Black Beans and Tomatoes:

- Add black beans, diced tomatoes (with juices), diced red bell pepper, and corn kernels to the pot. Stir to combine.

5. Pour Vegetable Broth:

- Pour in vegetable broth and bring the mixture to a simmer.

6. Simmer and Cook:

- Reduce heat to low, cover the pot, and let the chili simmer for 20-25 minutes or until the sweet potatoes are fork-tender.

7. Adjust Seasonings:

Taste and adjust the seasonings, adding more salt and pepper if necessary.

8. Serve

- Ladle the black bean and sweet potato chili into bowls.
- Garnish with fresh cilantro and avocado slices (if using).
- Serve with lime wedges on the side for squeezing.

Enjoy this hearty and nutritious black bean and sweet potato chili on its own or with a side of crusty bread or rice.

Note:

- Customize the spice level by adjusting the amount of chili powder and jalapeño.
- Feel free to add other vegetables like bell peppers, zucchini, or spinach for extra flavor and nutrition.
- This chili can be prepared in advance and reheated for a quick and satisfying meal.

Mediterranean Stuffed Peppers Recipe

Savor the flavors of the Mediterranean with these delicious stuffed peppers. Packed with a wholesome mixture of quinoa, vegetables, and Mediterranean herbs, these stuffed peppers are a nutritious and satisfying addition to your heart-healthy recipes.

Ingredients:

For the Stuffed Peppers:

- 4 Bell Peppers, halved and seeds removed
- 1 cup Quinoa, rinsed
- 2 cups Vegetable Broth
- 1 can (15 oz) Chickpeas, drained and rinsed
- 1 cup Cherry Tomatoes, halved
- 1/2 cup Kalamata Olives, sliced
- 1/2 cup Red Onion, finely chopped
- 1/2 cup Feta Cheese, crumbled

- 2 tablespoons Fresh Parsley, chopped

- 2 tablespoons Fresh Mint, chopped

- 3 tablespoons Olive Oil

- Salt and Pepper to taste

For the Mediterranean Dressing:

- 1/4 cup Olive Oil

- 2 tablespoons Red Wine Vinegar

- 1 teaspoon Dijon Mustard

- 1 clove Garlic, minced

- 1 teaspoon Honey or Maple Syrup

- Salt and Pepper to taste

Instructions:

1. Preheat the Oven:

- Preheat the oven to 375°F (190°C).

2. Prepare Quinoa:

- In a saucepan, combine quinoa and vegetable broth. Bring to a boil, then reduce heat, cover, and simmer for 15-20 minutes or until quinoa is cooked and liquid is absorbed. Fluff with a fork and set aside.

3. Roast Bell Peppers:

- Place the halved bell peppers in a baking dish.
- Drizzle olive oil over the peppers and season with salt and pepper.
- Roast in the preheated oven for 15-20 minutes or until the peppers are slightly tender.

4. Make Mediterranean Dressing:

- In a small bowl, whisk together olive oil, red wine vinegar, Dijon mustard, minced garlic, honey or maple syrup, salt, and pepper. Set aside.

5. Prepare Filling:

- In a large bowl, combine cooked quinoa, chickpeas, cherry tomatoes, Kalamata olives, red onion, feta cheese, fresh parsley, and fresh mint.

6. Combine with Dressing:

- Pour the Mediterranean dressing over the quinoa mixture and toss everything together until well combined.

7. Stuff the Peppers:

- Spoon the quinoa mixture into the roasted bell peppers, pressing down gently to pack the filling.

8. Bake:

- Return the stuffed peppers to the oven and bake for an additional 15-20 minutes or until the peppers are tender, and the filling is heated through.

9. Garnish and Serve:

- Garnish the stuffed peppers with additional fresh herbs.
- Serve warm, and enjoy the Mediterranean flavors in every bite.

Note:

- You can customize the filling by adding ingredients like artichoke hearts, cucumber, or roasted red peppers for added variety.
- Adjust the dressing ingredients to suit your taste preferences, adding more or less of specific herbs or spices.
- These stuffed peppers make for a delightful and colorful main course or a flavorful side dish for any Mediterranean-inspired meal.

Sides and Snacks

Garlic-Roasted Brussels Sprouts Recipe

Transform Brussels sprouts into a flavorful and irresistible side dish with this simple garlic-roasted Brussels sprouts recipe. The combination of roasted Brussels sprouts with garlic creates a deliciously savory dish that is both easy to make and delightful to the taste buds.

Ingredients:

- 1 pound Brussels Sprouts, trimmed and halved
- 3 tablespoons Olive Oil
- 4 cloves Garlic, minced
- Salt and Pepper to taste
- 1-2 tablespoons Balsamic Vinegar (optional, for drizzling)
- Grated Parmesan Cheese (optional, for serving)

Instructions:

1. Preheat the Oven:

- Preheat your oven to 400°F (200°C).

2. Prepare Brussels Sprouts:

- Trim the ends of the Brussels sprouts and cut them in half.

3. Toss with Olive Oil and Garlic:

- In a bowl, toss the Brussels sprouts with olive oil and minced garlic until they are evenly coated.

4. Season:

- Season the Brussels sprouts with salt and pepper to taste. Toss again to ensure even seasoning.

5. Spread on Baking Sheet:

- Spread the Brussels sprouts in a single layer on a baking sheet.

6. Roast in the Oven:

- Roast in the preheated oven for 20-25 minutes or until the Brussels sprouts are golden brown and crispy on the edges. Toss them halfway through the roasting time for even cooking.

7. Optional Drizzle with Balsamic Vinegar:

- If desired, drizzle balsamic vinegar over the roasted Brussels sprouts for added flavor. Toss to coat.

8. Serve:

- Transfer the garlic-roasted Brussels sprouts to a serving dish.

9. Optional Parmesan Cheese:

- If you like, sprinkle grated Parmesan cheese over the Brussels sprouts before serving.
- Serve the garlic-roasted Brussels sprouts immediately as a delightful and flavorful side dish.

Note:

- Customize the seasoning by adding additional herbs or spices such as thyme, rosemary, or red pepper flakes.
- Adjust the roasting time based on the size of the Brussels sprouts and your desired level of crispiness.
- Experiment with different drizzles such as lemon juice or honey for a unique twist.

Spiced Chickpea Snack Mix Recipe

Enjoy a crunchy and flavorful snack with this spiced chickpea snack mix. Roasted chickpeas combined with a mix of nuts and seeds create a satisfying and nutritious snack that's perfect for any occasion.

Ingredients:

- 2 cans (15 oz each) Chickpeas, drained and rinsed
- 1 cup Mixed Nuts (almonds, cashews, walnuts, etc.)
- 1/2 cup Pumpkin Seeds (Pepitas)
- 1/2 cup Sunflower Seeds
- 2 tablespoons Olive Oil

- 1 teaspoon Ground Cumin

- 1 teaspoon Paprika

- 1/2 teaspoon Ground Coriander

- 1/2 teaspoon Garlic Powder

- 1/4 teaspoon Cayenne Pepper (adjust to taste)

- Salt to taste

Instructions:

1. Preheat the Oven:

- Preheat your oven to 400°F (200°C).

2. Prepare Chickpeas:

- Drain and rinse the chickpeas. Pat them dry with a paper towel to remove excess moisture.

3. Roast Chickpeas:

- Place the chickpeas on a baking sheet in a single layer.

- Bake in the preheated oven for 20-25 minutes or until the chickpeas are crispy. Shake the baking sheet occasionally for even roasting.

4. Prepare Nut and Seed Mix:

- In a large bowl, combine mixed nuts, pumpkin seeds, and sunflower seeds.

5. Spice Mixture:

- In a small bowl, mix together olive oil, ground cumin, paprika, ground coriander, garlic powder, cayenne pepper, and salt.

6. Toss and Coat:

- Pour the spice mixture over the nut and seed mix. Toss until everything is well coated.

7. Combine with Chickpeas:

- Once the chickpeas are roasted and crispy, add them to the nut and seed mix. Toss everything together until evenly combined.

8. Serve or Cool:

- Allow the spiced chickpea snack mix to cool before serving.
- Enjoy this flavorful and crunchy snack mix on its own or as a topping for salads and yogurt.

Note:

- Feel free to customize the spice blend to suit your taste preferences. Add more or less cayenne pepper for heat, or experiment with your favorite spices.

- This spiced chickpea snack mix can be stored in an airtight container for several days, making it a convenient and tasty snack option.

Guilt-Free Sweet Potato Fries Recipe

Indulge in a healthier alternative to traditional fries with these guilt-free sweet potato fries. Baked to perfection and seasoned with a delightful blend of spices, these sweet potato fries are not only delicious but also a nutritious addition to your heart-conscious snacks.

Ingredients:

- 2 large Sweet Potatoes, peeled and cut into matchsticks or wedges
- 2 tablespoons Olive Oil
- 1 teaspoon Smoked Paprika
- 1/2 teaspoon Garlic Powder
- 1/2 teaspoon Onion Powder
- 1/2 teaspoon Ground Cumin
- 1/2 teaspoon Chili Powder
- Salt and Pepper to taste
- Fresh Parsley, chopped (for garnish, optional)

Instructions:

1. Preheat the Oven:

- Preheat your oven to 425°F (220°C).

2. Prepare Sweet Potatoes:

- Peel the sweet potatoes and cut them into matchsticks or wedges, ensuring they are of similar size for even baking.

3. Coat with Olive Oil and Spices:

- In a large bowl, toss the sweet potato matchsticks or wedges with olive oil until evenly coated.
- In a separate bowl, mix together smoked paprika, garlic powder, onion powder, ground cumin, chili powder, salt, and pepper.

4. Season Sweet Potatoes:

- Sprinkle the spice mixture over the sweet potatoes and toss until they are well coated with the spices.

5. Arrange on Baking Sheet:

- Spread the seasoned sweet potatoes in a single layer on a baking sheet, ensuring they have some space between them for even crisping.

6. Bake in the Oven:

- Bake in the preheated oven for 20-25 minutes, flipping the sweet potatoes halfway through the baking time, or until they are golden brown and crispy.

7. Garnish and Serve:

- Remove from the oven and garnish with chopped fresh parsley if desired.
- Serve these guilt-free sweet potato fries immediately as a tasty and nutritious snack or side dish.

Note:

- Feel free to adjust the seasoning to suit your taste preferences. Experiment with different herbs and spices for variety.
- For extra crispiness, you can place a wire rack on the baking sheet to allow air circulation around the sweet potato fries.
- Pair these guilt-free sweet potato fries with a light yogurt-based dip or your favorite salsa for added flavor.

Desserts with Heart

Berry-licious Yogurt Parfait Recipe

Indulge in a delightful and healthy treat with this berry-licious yogurt parfait. Layered with creamy yogurt, fresh berries, and a crunchy granola topping, this parfait is not only delicious but also a nutritious option for a heart-conscious snack or breakfast.

Ingredients:

- 1 cup Greek Yogurt (plain or flavored)
- 1 cup Mixed Berries (strawberries, blueberries, raspberries, etc.)
- 1/2 cup Granola
- 1 tablespoon Honey or Maple Syrup (optional, for drizzling)
- Fresh Mint Leaves (for garnish, optional)

Instructions:

1. Prepare the Berries:

- Wash and prepare the mixed berries. Slice strawberries if using.

2. Layer the Yogurt:

- In a glass or a bowl, start with a layer of Greek yogurt at the bottom.

3. Add a Layer of Berries:

- Add a layer of mixed berries on top of the yogurt.

4. Sprinkle Granola:

- Sprinkle a layer of granola over the berries. Choose your favorite granola variety, such as nutty, honey, or vanilla-flavored.

5. Repeat the Layers:

- Repeat the layers until the glass or bowl is filled, ending with a layer of berries on top.

6. Drizzle with Honey or Maple Syrup:

- Drizzle honey or maple syrup over the top for a touch of sweetness (optional).

7. Garnish with Fresh Mint:

- Garnish with fresh mint leaves for a burst of freshness and a hint of aroma (optional).

8. Serve and Enjoy:

- Serve the berry-licious yogurt parfait immediately and enjoy the layers of flavors and textures.

Note:

- Feel free to customize the parfait with your favorite fruits, such as sliced bananas, kiwi, or mango.
- Experiment with different types of yogurt, including flavored or non-dairy options like almond or coconut yogurt.
- Adjust the sweetness level by adding more or less honey or maple syrup according to your taste preferences.
- This yogurt parfait is not only a delicious breakfast option but also makes for a refreshing and satisfying snack.

Dark Chocolate Avocado Mousse Recipe

Indulge in a rich and creamy dessert that also packs a nutritional punch with this dark chocolate avocado mousse. Silky smooth and decadently chocolatey, this mousse is not only delicious but also a heart-healthy treat.

Ingredients:

- 2 ripe Avocados, peeled and pitted
- 1/2 cup Dark Chocolate Chips or chopped Dark Chocolate (at least 70% cocoa)
- 1/4 cup Unsweetened Cocoa Powder
- 1/4 cup Maple Syrup or Agave Nectar
- 1 teaspoon Vanilla Extract
- 1/4 teaspoon Salt

- Fresh Berries or Mint Leaves (for garnish, optional)

Instructions:

1. Melt Chocolate:

- In a heatproof bowl, melt the dark chocolate chips or chopped dark chocolate. You can use a microwave or a double boiler for this. Allow it to cool slightly.

2. Blend Avocados:

- In a blender or food processor, combine the ripe avocados, melted chocolate, unsweetened cocoa powder, maple syrup or agave nectar, vanilla extract, and salt.

3. Blend Until Smooth:

- Blend the ingredients until you achieve a smooth and creamy consistency. Scrape down the sides of the blender or processor as needed.

4. Chill the Mousse:

- Transfer the chocolate avocado mixture to a bowl or individual serving glasses.
- Cover and refrigerate for at least 2 hours or until the mousse is nicely chilled.

5. Serve and Garnish:

- Once chilled, serve the dark chocolate avocado mousse in bowls or glasses.
- Garnish with fresh berries or mint leaves if desired.
- Indulge in this luscious and guilt-free dark chocolate avocado mousse.

Note:

- Adjust the sweetness by adding more or less maple syrup or agave nectar according to your taste preferences.
- For an extra flavor boost, you can add a hint of espresso or coffee extract to the mousse.
- This dessert is not only a delicious standalone treat but also pairs well with a dollop of whipped coconut cream or a sprinkle of chopped nuts for added texture.

Fruit Salad with Mint-Lime Drizzle Recipe

Elevate the freshness of your fruit salad with a refreshing mint-lime drizzle. This simple yet vibrant dressing adds a burst of flavor to a colorful array of fruits, creating a delightful and healthy treat.

Ingredients:

For the Fruit Salad:

- 2 cups Watermelon, cubed

- 1 cup Strawberries, hulled and halved

- 1 cup Pineapple, diced

- 1 cup Grapes, halved

- 1 Mango, peeled and diced

- 1 Kiwi, peeled and sliced

- 1 Orange, peeled and segmented

- 1 Banana, sliced

- Fresh Mint Leaves (for garnish)

For the Mint-Lime Drizzle:

- 2 tablespoons Fresh Mint, finely chopped

- 2 tablespoons Lime Juice

- 1-2 tablespoons Honey or Agave Nectar (adjust to taste)

Instructions:

1. Prepare the Fruit:

- Wash, peel, and chop all the fruits as needed.

2. Arrange in a Bowl:

- In a large bowl, combine watermelon, strawberries, pineapple, grapes, mango, kiwi, orange segments, and banana. Gently toss to mix.

3. Prepare the Mint-Lime Drizzle:

- In a small bowl, whisk together finely chopped mint, lime juice, and honey or agave nectar. Adjust the sweetness according to your preference.

4. Drizzle over the Fruit:

- Drizzle the mint-lime dressing over the mixed fruits. Toss gently to coat the fruits evenly with the dressing.

5. Chill (Optional):

- If time allows, refrigerate the fruit salad for about 30 minutes to let the flavors meld and the salad to chill.

6. Garnish:

- Before serving, garnish the fruit salad with additional fresh mint leaves.

7. Serve:

- Serve the fruit salad with mint-lime drizzle as a refreshing and colorful dessert or snack.
- Enjoy the burst of flavors from the sweet and juicy fruits combined with the zesty mint-lime drizzle.

Note:

- Customize the fruit selection based on seasonal availability and your personal preferences.

- Experiment with additional herbs like basil or cilantro for a unique twist to the dressing.

- This fruit salad is a versatile dish that can be served on its own, as a side dish, or as a topping for yogurt or ice cream.

Beverages for Cardiovascular Bliss

Hibiscus Ginger Iced Tea Recipe

Quench your thirst with a refreshing and flavorful Hibiscus Ginger Iced Tea. This vibrant beverage combines the tartness of hibiscus with the warmth of ginger, creating a cooling drink that is perfect for hot days or as a delightful accompaniment to any meal.

Ingredients:

- 4 cups Water
- 3 Hibiscus Tea Bags
- 1 tablespoon Fresh Ginger, grated
- 1/4 cup Honey or Agave Nectar (adjust to taste)
- Ice Cubes
- Lemon slices or Mint leaves (for garnish, optional)

Instructions:

1. Boil Water:

- Bring 4 cups of water to a boil in a pot.

2. Steep Hibiscus Tea Bags:

- Once the water is boiling, remove it from heat. Add hibiscus tea bags to the hot water and steep for about 5-7 minutes. Adjust the steeping time based on your desired strength.

3. Add Grated Ginger:

- Grate fresh ginger and add it to the hot hibiscus tea. Allow it to steep along with the tea bags for an additional 5 minutes. Adjust the ginger quantity based on your preference for spiciness.

4. Sweeten the Tea:

- Stir in honey or agave nectar to sweeten the tea. Adjust the sweetness to your liking.

5. Strain and Chill:

- Remove the tea bags and grated ginger from the pot. Strain the tea to remove any remaining ginger particles.
- Allow the tea to cool to room temperature, and then refrigerate until chilled.

6. Serve Over Ice:

- Once the hibiscus ginger tea is chilled, fill glasses with ice cubes and pour the tea over the ice.

7. Garnish (Optional):

- Garnish the iced tea with lemon slices or mint leaves for an extra burst of freshness.

8. Stir and Enjoy:

- Stir the iced tea and enjoy the delightful combination of hibiscus and ginger flavors.

Note:

- You can experiment with the level of sweetness and adjust the honey or agave nectar accordingly.
- Feel free to add a splash of club soda for a fizzy variation of this hibiscus ginger iced tea.
- This tea can be made in larger batches and stored in the refrigerator for a quick and refreshing beverage anytime.

Berry Blast Smoothie Recipe

Start your day with a burst of fruity goodness with this Berry Blast Smoothie. Packed with a variety of berries, yogurt, and a touch of honey, this smoothie is not only delicious but also a nutritious way to kickstart your morning or refuel during the day.

Ingredients:

- 1 cup Mixed Berries (strawberries, blueberries, raspberries)
- 1/2 Banana, frozen
- 1/2 cup Greek Yogurt (plain or flavored)
- 1/2 cup Almond Milk (or any milk of your choice)
- 1 tablespoon Honey or Maple Syrup (adjust to taste)

- Ice Cubes (optional)

Instructions:

1. Prepare the Berries:

- If using fresh berries, wash them thoroughly. If using frozen berries, ensure they are properly thawed.

2. Combine Ingredients:

- In a blender, combine mixed berries, frozen banana, Greek yogurt, almond milk, and honey or maple syrup.

3. Blend Until Smooth:

- Blend the ingredients until you achieve a smooth and creamy consistency. If the smoothie is too thick, you can add more almond milk to reach your desired consistency.

4. Taste and Adjust:

- Taste the smoothie and adjust the sweetness by adding more honey or maple syrup if needed.

5. Add Ice Cubes (Optional):

- If you prefer a colder and frostier texture, add a handful of ice cubes to the blender and blend again until smooth.

6. Pour and Serve:

- Pour the Berry Blast Smoothie into a glass.

7. Garnish (Optional):

- Garnish with additional berries or a slice of banana on the rim of the glass for a decorative touch.

8. Enjoy:

- Sip and enjoy the refreshing and nutrient-packed goodness of the Berry Blast Smoothie.

Note:

- Feel free to customize the smoothie by adding other fruits such as mango, pineapple, or kiwi.
- For an extra protein boost, consider adding a scoop of protein powder or a tablespoon of chia seeds.
- This smoothie is not only a great breakfast option but also a fantastic snack for any time of the day.

Infused Water Creations Recipes

Stay hydrated and add a burst of natural flavor to your water with these refreshing infused water creations. These combinations are not only delicious but also a healthy and enjoyable way to stay on top of your hydration game.

1. Citrus Mint Splash:

Ingredients:

- 1 Lemon, sliced

- 1 Lime, sliced

- 1 Orange, sliced

- Fresh Mint Leaves

Instructions:

- Combine lemon, lime, and orange slices in a pitcher.

- Add fresh mint leaves.

- Fill the pitcher with water and refrigerate for a few hours before serving.

2. Cucumber Basil Bliss:

Ingredients:

- 1/2 Cucumber, sliced

- Fresh Basil Leaves

Instructions:

- Place cucumber slices and fresh basil leaves in a pitcher.

- Add water and let it infuse in the refrigerator for a couple of hours.

3. Berry Melon Medley:

Ingredients:

- 1 cup Mixed Berries (strawberries, blueberries, raspberries)

- 1 cup Watermelon, cubed
- 1 cup Cantaloupe, cubed

Instructions:

- Combine mixed berries, watermelon, and cantaloupe in a pitcher.
- Fill with water and let it infuse for a refreshing fruity blend.

4. Pineapple Coconut Splash:

Ingredients:

- 1 cup Pineapple, chunks
- 1/2 cup Coconut Water
- 1 Lime, sliced

Instructions:

- Place pineapple chunks and lime slices in a pitcher.
- Add coconut water and regular water. Allow it to infuse in the refrigerator.

5. Apple Cinnamon Infusion:

Ingredients:

- 1 Apple, thinly sliced
- 2 Cinnamon Sticks

Instructions:

- Combine apple slices and cinnamon sticks in a pitcher.
- Add water and let it infuse, creating a subtly sweet and spicy concoction.

6. Ginger Lemon Elixir:

Ingredients:

- 1 Lemon, sliced
- 1-2 inches Fresh Ginger, thinly sliced

Instructions:

- Place lemon slices and ginger in a pitcher.
- Fill with water and let it infuse for a zesty and invigorating drink.

7. Raspberry Rose Refresher:

Ingredients:

- 1 cup Raspberries
- 1-2 teaspoons Rose Water (edible)

Instructions:

- Combine raspberries and rose water in a pitcher.
- Fill with water and let it infuse for a delicate and fragrant beverage.

Instructions for All:

- For best results, let the infused water creations sit in the refrigerator for at least 2-4 hours, or overnight for a more intense flavor.
- You can refill the pitcher with water a few times before replacing the fruits and herbs for continued enjoyment.
- Feel free to get creative and mix and match ingredients to find your favorite combinations!

Conclusion

In the journey toward optimal health, embracing a heart-healthy lifestyle becomes a pivotal choice—one that resonates through every aspect of our well-being. As we navigate the intricate connection between our dietary choices and cardiovascular health, "Heart healthy cookbook for all: Easy Delicious, Low Fat, Low Sodium Heart Healthy Recipes" stands as a guide, inviting you to savor the symphony of flavors that nourish both body and soul.

Understanding the vital importance of heart-friendly eating forms the cornerstone of this culinary exploration. By delving into the foundations of heart-healthy cuisine and comprehending the intricacies of cardiovascular wellness, you gain not just knowledge but a roadmap for conscious and healthful living.

The heart of this culinary journey beats in the kitchens, where the symphony of ingredients comes to life. From energizing morning smoothies that awaken your senses to nutrient-packed oatmeal variations that fuel your day, each recipe is a celebration of wholesome goodness. The introduction of hearty soups, vibrant salads, and satisfying main courses illustrates that heart-healthy eating is not about sacrifice but about reveling in the abundance of nature's bounty.

Recognizing that snacks play a crucial role in our culinary narrative, "Heart healthy cookbook for all" introduces guilt-free sweet potato fries, spiced chickpea snack mix, and a decadent dark chocolate avocado mousse. These treats redefine the notion of indulgence, offering satisfaction without compromising on your commitment to heart health.

Infused water creations emerge as refreshing companions on this journey, reminding us that hydration can be a delightfully flavorful experience. As you sip on these natural elixirs, you infuse your body with the vitality of fruits, herbs, and spices, promoting a wholesome approach to nourishment.

"Heart healthy cookbook for all" is more than a collection of recipes; it's an invitation to savor the artistry of wholesome cooking, to revel in the joy of mindful eating, and to celebrate the vibrancy of a heart-healthy life. Each recipe is a page in the culinary story of well-being, inviting you to partake in the symphony of flavors that harmonize to create a healthier, more vibrant you. May your heart be nourished, and your culinary journey be filled with joy and abundance. Cheers to a vibrant heart and a life well-lived!

www.ingramcontent.com/pod-product-compliance
Lightning Source LLC
Chambersburg PA
CBHW070833260726
48660CB00005B/2040